MASTECTOMY RECOVERY COOKBOOK

Complete Guide Unlocking The Secrets Of Nutrition To Rapid Healing After Surgery Success, Nourishing Meal Plans, Recipes, Tips For Optimal Health Wellness)

DR. ALLAN FREDA

Contents

The book includes a lot of information, like meal plans, healing foods, and expert advice to help with long-term health. This cookbook is very helpful for learning about the specific food needs and problems that people who have had mastectomy surgery face. It talks about how important diet is for healing and gives useful tips on how to feed the body well during this very important time. Designed to help people heal and improve their general health, the Mastectomy Recovery Cookbook is a reliable guide for those on their way to recovery.

THE BEGINNING

A mastectomy, in which one or both breasts are surgically removed, is an important part of treating breast cancer. During the recovery time, people often have physical and emotional problems. It can be hard to get better after having a mastectomy because you have to go through physical rehabilitation, get mental support, and change what you eat. The Mastectomy Recovery Cookbook is meant to be a complete guide to this time after surgery, with a focus on good nutrition.

It includes meal plans, healing recipes, and health tips from experts for long-term success.

This cookbook talks about how important nutrition is for recovery. It has useful tips and tasty recipes that are designed to help with healing, give you more energy, and improve your general health.

About getting a mastectomy and healing

A mastectomy is a surgery that is mostly used to treat breast cancer. It includes taking out breast tissue and, in some cases, lymph nodes that are close by. As much as a mastectomy can save lives, it can also be very hard on the person having it, both physically and emotionally. Many things need to be done to recover from a mastectomy, such as wound healing, pain management, rehabilitation exercises, emotional support, and changes to food.

The recovery time can be different for each person, based on things like the extent of the surgery, their health, and how strong they are in general.

It's important to look at mastectomy recovery as a whole, taking into account not only the physical needs but also the mental and nutritional ones of the person. During the recovery process, good nutrition is very important for helping the body heal, boosting the immune system, managing side effects, and promoting general health.

Understanding Why Nutrition Is Important After a Mastectomy

What you eat is very important for healing after a mastectomy. To keep tissues healthy, the immune system strong, inflammation under control, and general health and vitality high, the body needs certain nutrients.

A good diet can help with common problems that come up after surgery, like feeling tired, sick, or unable to go to the toilet.

It can also lower the risk of complications and speed up the healing process.

But surgery can change your hunger, digestion, and ability to absorb nutrients, so it's important to be very careful about what you eat while you're healing.

A healthy, well-balanced diet full of protein, vitamins, minerals, antioxidants, and other nutrients is important for healing and improving general health. Also, some nutrients and foods may help people who have recently had a mastectomy in certain ways, like helping tissues heal, lowering inflammation, and keeping hormones in balance.

Important Things to Think About When Eating After a Mastectomy

For the best healing after a mastectomy, there are a few important nutritional things to keep in mind.

A healthy diet should include enough protein to help fix tissues and heal wounds, water to keep the body's fluid balance and support cell function, fiber to keep you from getting constipated and improve digestive health, and antioxidants to lower inflammation and help the immune system work.

To make sure the body gets all the nutrients it needs, it's also important to eat a wide range of nutrient-dense foods, such as fruits, veggies, whole grains, lean proteins, and healthy fats.

Along with macronutrients and vitamins, it's important to pay attention to your hydration levels. Staying hydrated is good for your health and helps your body get rid of toxins.

Eating foods like fatty fish, flaxseeds, and walnuts that are high in omega-3 fatty acids may also help lower inflammation and improve heart health, which is especially important while you are healing.

Planning meals for the best recovery

Planning meals is an important part of recovering from a mastectomy because it makes sure that people have access to healthy, easy-to-find foods that help them heal and stay healthy.

When planning your meals after having a mastectomy, it's important to focus on foods that are high in vitamins, minerals, and antioxidants.

This could mean eating a wide range of colorful fruits and veggies, lean proteins like chicken, fish, tofu, and beans, whole grains like brown rice, quinoa, and oats, and healthy fats from foods like nuts, avocados, and olive oil.

Adding herbs, spices, and sauces to meals can also make them taste better and give you more options without lowering their nutritional value.

Planning meals ahead of time can also help people deal with tiredness, keep up their energy, and avoid nutritional deficiencies by making sure they have access to healthy, filling meals throughout the day.

Recipes that will help you heal after having a mastectomy

Healing recipes designed to help with recovery after a mastectomy can give you food, warmth, and fun while you're getting better. These recipes are mostly about using healthy foods that are high in nutrients, like anti-inflammatory foods, immune-boosting foods, and foods that are full of vitamins, minerals, and antioxidants.

Healing recipes might include different kinds of soups, stews, salads, smoothies, and healthy snacks that are simple to digest, easy on the stomach, and full of important nutrients. Adding herbs, spices, and culinary herbs that are known to have healing qualities can also make food taste better and be healthier without adding too much salt, sugar, or unhealthy fats.

Healing recipes can give people a wide range of tastes, textures, and colors, making their eating experience more interesting and rewarding while also helping them on their way to recovery.

Advice from experts on how to stay healthy after a mastectomy

Along with tactics that focus on nutrition, several expert tips can help with long-term health after a mastectomy. Some of these are getting regular exercise to improve strength, flexibility, and heart health; dealing with stress through mindfulness, meditation, and deep breathing exercises; getting help from doctors, counselors, or support groups to deal with emotional needs and concerns; and making time for self-care activities that make you happy, relax, and improve your overall health.

It's also important to know about follow-up care, keep an eye out for signs of recurrence or complications, and talk to your healthcare providers regularly to address any questions or concerns that may come up during your healing. People can improve their health, vitality, and quality of life in the long run by taking a holistic approach to recovery after a mastectomy.

Disclaimer

The information in this book is for informational purposes only and should not replace professional medical advice, diagnosis, or treatment. Always consult your physician or a qualified health provider regarding any medical concerns. Do not disregard professional medical advice or delay seeking it based on information in this book.

The author does not endorse or have affiliations with any mentioned entities. References are for informational purposes only.

Consult your healthcare provider before making dietary or lifestyle changes, especially during recovery from surgery, as individual needs vary.

Results may vary, and the information provided is not guaranteed to produce specific outcomes.

By reading this book, you acknowledge and agree to consult your healthcare provider before implementing any information herein.

For further guidance, consult your healthcare provider or reputable medical websites for reliable information on surgery recovery diets.

CHAPTER 1
FEEDING THE BASICS

Getting through the rehab process after a mastectomy means paying close attention to both your physical and nutritional needs. At this point, you need to have a full understanding of how your food affects your recovery and health in general.

In the parts that follow, we'll talk about the basics of nutrition. These will include everything from understanding your nutritional needs during recovery to making sure your kitchen has all the tools and equipment you need to make healing meals.

Figuring Out What Your Body Needs for Recovery:

Recovery from a mastectomy is a very important time that needs extra attention to nutrition needs. During this time, the body goes through a lot of changes.

A good diet is very important for healing, boosting the immune system, and getting back to full health. As they heal from mastectomy surgery, some people may feel tired, lose their appetite, get sick, or change the way they like their food.

So, it's important to make sure that the food fits these issues while still giving the best nutrition.

Protein is important for repairing tissues and building muscle strength, which are both very important for healing after surgery. Getting protein from lean sources like chicken, fish, tofu, beans, and dairy can help you meet these goals. Eating lots of foods that are high in vitamins, minerals, and antioxidants can also help your immune system and fight inflammation, which speeds up the healing process.

Also, staying properly hydrated is very important for your health and healing as a whole.

Drinking a lot of water throughout the day keeps you from becoming dehydrated, helps the body get rid of toxins, and supports the functions of cells.

Herbal teas, fruit-infused water, and broths are some other drinks that can help you stay hydrated and provide extra nutrients and healing effects.

It's just as important to know about each person's dietary needs or restrictions during the recovery process. Some people may need to make changes, like staying away from foods that interact badly with their medications or make digestive problems worse. Talking to a trained dietitian or health care provider can help you get personalised advice that fits your needs and get the most out of your nutrition while you're recovering.

Putting together a kitchen that works:

A well-stocked kitchen makes it easier to make healthy meals that help the healing process. Putting healthy foods in your kitchen makes it easy to get the nutrients you need and makes it easier to make meals that are both balanced and good for you. When preparing your kitchen for healing after a mastectomy, you might want to include the following essentials:

1. Whole Grains: Choose whole grains like brown rice, quinoa, oats, and whole wheat pasta to fill you up and give you fiber to keep your digestive system healthy.

2. Fresh Food: Put a bunch of different colored fruits and veggies in your fridge. They are full of vitamins, minerals, and antioxidants. Leafy greens, berries, citrus fruits, cruciferous veggies, and other foods that are high in nutrients can help your immune system and your health in general.

3. Lean Proteins: To help repair muscles and feel full, choose lean protein sources like skinless chicken, fish, eggs, beans, tofu, and low-fat dairy products.

4. Healthy Fats: To keep your heart healthy and help your body absorb nutrients better, eat foods

like bananas, nuts, seeds, olive oil, and fatty fish like salmon.

5. Herbs and Spices: Try using different herbs and spices to give your food more flavor and depth without adding too much salt or unhealthy sauces. A lot of herbs and spices, like rosemary, basil, thyme, and turmeric, can be used in cooking and as medicine.

6. Healing Ingredients: Use certain ingredients that are known to help the body heal, like ginger for sickness, garlic to boost the immune system, and honey to soothe sore throats or dry coughs.

By having these things in your home, you can make it easier to make meals, make sure you have access to healthy foods, and give yourself the power to make healthier choices while you're recovering.

Important tools and equipment for cooking:

Having the right cooking tools and equipment can make making meals easier and more efficient in the kitchen, especially while you're recovering and your energy may be all over the place.

Buying good cooking essentials makes them easier to use and lets people focus on feeding themselves without having to deal with extra stress or frustration. Take a look at these important cooking tools and equipment for recovering from a mastectomy:

1. Non-Stick Cookware: Pots and pans that don't stick let you cook with less oil or fat, which makes cooking healthier and cleaning up easy.

Pick durable, non-toxic cookware that spreads heat evenly and can handle a lot of use.

2. Sharp Knives: Making sure you have a set of sharp, comfortable knives is important for cutting, chopping, and slicing food safely and accurately. Not only do dull knives make things harder to do, but they also raise the risk of accidents, especially for people who are weak or have trouble moving their hands.

3. Cutting Boards: To prepare food on a stable surface, buy cutting boards that are made of wood, bamboo, or plastic that will last. Having more than one cutting board lets you keep raw meats, poultry, fruits, and veggies separate, which lowers the chance of cross-contamination.

4. Blender or Food Processor: You can make smoothies, soups, sauces, and purees with a blender or food processor. This makes it easier to eat healthy foods in a form that your body can handle. For ease of use, look for models with speed levels that you can change and parts that are easy to clean.

5. A slow cooker or an instant pot are multifunctional tools that make cooking easier by letting you make hearty stews, soups, and one-pot meals without having to touch the food. Their time-saving and customizable features are especially helpful for people who are tired or have trouble moving around.

6. Combining Bowls and Utensils: You need a set of mixing bowls in different sizes and tools like spatulas, whisks, and ladles to mix materials, stir them, and serve the food. Choose designs that are light, well-balanced, and easy to hold for long amounts of time.

7. Containers for Storage: To store leftovers, meal-prepped ingredients, and batch-cooked meals, buy a variety of containers that are BPA-free and have lids that fit securely. Keeping food in the right way helps it stay fresh, cuts down on waste, and makes it easier to control portions.

8. Kitchen Scale: A digital kitchen scale gives you exact measurements for controlling portions and following recipes, which is especially helpful when you are following certain meal plans or dietary advice. It helps make sure that the amounts of ingredients and nutritional information are always the same.

9. Oven Mitts and Pot Holders: Heat-resistant oven mitts and pot holders keep your hands and surfaces safe from damage caused by heat. When handling hot cookware or bakeware, choose choices that are long-lasting, insulated, and give you a good grip and enough coverage.

Getting these important cooking tools and equipment for your home will make making meals easier, safer, and more efficient, so you can focus on eating well while you're recovering from a mastectomy.

CHAPTER 2
BREAKFAST RECIPES THAT HEAL

Nutrition is a very important part of getting better after having a mastectomy. It helps the body heal and improves general health.

Many people say that breakfast is the most important meal of the day because it sets the tone for the rest of the day's food.

This part of the Mastectomy Recovery Cookbook is all about healthy and comfortable breakfast ideas that are designed to help with recovery after surgery.

This complete guide aims to provide a wide range of healing recipes, including energizing smoothies and juices, comforting porridges and oats, and protein-rich breakfast meals so that people in recovery can find something that works for them.

Smoothies and juices are great for breakfast while you're recovering from a mastectomy because they are easy to swallow, full of nutrients, and can be made with ingredients that help you heal and give you more energy.

Putting different kinds of fruits and veggies into juices and smoothies gives your body vitamins, minerals, antioxidants, and water, all of which help it heal. Leafy veggies, berries, citrus fruits, ginger, and turmeric are all very good for you because they reduce inflammation and boost the immune system.

Adding protein sources like Greek yogurt, nut butter, or plant-based protein powder also makes you feel fuller and helps your muscles heal. Adding healthy fats from things like flaxseed oil or avocado helps the body absorb nutrients even better and gives you energy all morning. You can have these energizing smoothies and drinks for breakfast on their own, or you can pair them with other healthy recipes for a more complete meal.

Warm muesli and porridge

Oats and porridge are traditional breakfast foods that are known for being comforting and healthy. This makes them great choices for people who are healing from mastectomy surgery.

Not only are these foods easy to handle, but they also have a lot of fiber, which is good for your digestive health and helps keep your blood sugar levels steady, giving you energy all day.

By adding rolled oats, quinoa, chia seeds, and flaxseeds to cereal, you can change the texture, and taste, and get extra nutrients like protein and omega-3 fatty acids.

Not only does adding vegetables, nuts, seeds, and a drizzle of honey or maple syrup to porridge make it taste better, but it also makes it healthier.

People who have to follow certain diets or just don't like dairy can easily change the taste of porridge by adding different grains like buckwheat or millet and non-dairy milk like almond milk or oat milk. Porridges and oats are soothing and filling breakfast foods that can be eaten hot or cold. They help the body heal and are good for general health.

Breakfast Dishes Full of Protein

For the body to heal after a mastectomy, protein is very important because it helps fix tissues, keep the immune system healthy, and build muscle.

Adding breakfast foods that are high in protein to the recovery diet helps meet the body's higher protein needs and promotes the best possible recovery results. Eggs, tofu, lean meats, fish, and legumes are all great sources of high-quality protein that can be used in several different breakfast meals. There are a lot of different ways to make protein-rich breakfast foods that are both tasty and good for you.

Some examples are omelets, frittatas, breakfast bowls, and breakfast wraps. Combining protein sources with complex carbs like whole grains, veggies, and fruits helps keep blood sugar levels steady and gives you energy all morning.

Adding healthy fats from foods like avocado, nuts, and seeds also makes food taste better and makes you feel full. People who are recovering from a mastectomy can help their muscles heal, keep their energy up, and improve their general nutrition by choosing breakfast foods that are high in protein. This will make their recovery go more smoothly and effectively.

 food is an important part of the diet for recovering from a mastectomy because it gives you energy, comfort, and nutrients that you need while you heal. People who are healing from surgery can choose from a wide range of foods, including energizing smoothies and juices, comforting porridges and oats, and protein-packed breakfast dishes.

People can nourish their bodies, help them recover better, and maintain long-term health and energy by making these healing recipes a part of their daily lives.

CHAPTER 3
MAKING SOUPS AND BREADS LAST LONGER

When recovering from a mastectomy, diet is very important for helping the body heal and get healthy again. When it comes to food choices, soups, and broths stand out as gentle but effective ways to get the nutrition you need after surgery.

These liquid foods are full of important nutrients, easy to stomach, and pleasant to taste. They are comforting during a time of physical change and healing. As you read this, we'll dive into the world of healing soups and broths, looking at their many forms and focusing on how they can help with cancer recovery.

Rich in nutrients vegetable soups

After having a mastectomy, vegetable soups are an important part of a healthy diet. These soups are full of fiber, vitamins, minerals, antioxidants, and other nutrients that the body needs to mend tissues and keep the immune system strong.

Adding a variety of veggies, like bell peppers, carrots, spinach, kale, broccoli, and spinach, guarantees a wide range of nutrients that are good for your health as a whole. Adding herbs and spices to soups not only makes them taste better but also gives them anti-inflammatory and antimicrobial qualities that help the body heal even more. Vegetable soups are a tasty and healthy way to help your body recover and feel better, whether you eat them for lunch or as a cozy dinner.

Broths Full of Protein

Protein is an important food for healing after surgery because it helps cells grow, wounds heal, and the immune system work. Especially broths made from high-quality meats like chicken, beef, or fish are great ways to get protein in a form that the body can easily digest and use. Simmering animal bones, cartilage, and connective tissue for a long time not only gets rid of waste but also releases healing chemicals like collagen and gelatin that help keep joints healthy and skin flexible.

In addition, the gentle warmth of soup helps the body heal by soothing sore muscles and relieving digestive pain. By adding protein-rich broths to their post-mastectomy diet, people can make sure they get enough food to help them heal and get stronger.

Bone broths and stocks that heal

As powerful elixirs for mastectomy recovery, bone broths, and stocks are known for their unmatched healing and therapeutic benefits. These elixirs are made by slowly simmering a mix of bones from chicken, beef, fish, and aromatic veggies and herbs.

They are high in minerals, amino acids, collagen, and gelatin, all of which are important for healing and regenerating tissue. When it comes to helping the body heal, collagen is especially helpful because it strengthens connective tissues, makes skin more elastic, and keeps joints healthy.

Bone broths also have gelatin in them, which helps the gut heal and process by reducing inflammation and protecting the lining of the digestive tract. Healing bone broths and stocks are great for people who are trying to get healthy again after having a mastectomy. They can be drunk on their own or used as a base for filling soups and stews. People can start a path of healing and renewal by accepting the healing power of these liquid treasures. Each soothing sip can nourish both the body and the soul.

CHAPTER 4
MAIN COURSES FOR EVERYONE

Making sure you eat healthy foods while you're recovering from a mastectomy is very important for your health and healing. The idea of wholesome main courses goes beyond just giving you food; it includes giving your body nutrient-rich foods that help you heal, boost your immune system, and keep you healthy in the long run.

This part of the mastectomy recovery cookbook goes into more detail about the different types of main courses that can be made to fit different dietary needs and tastes.

Chicken and turkey dishes with lots of flavor:
People who have recently had a mastectomy may benefit greatly from eating lean meats like chicken and turkey while they are healing.

These chicken options are not only high in high-quality protein, which is needed to repair tissues, but they also have many important nutrients, such as iron, zinc, and B vitamins. In this part of the guide, the focus is on making tasty meals that meet nutritional needs and please the taste buds.

The recipes here are designed to help you eat well and have fun while you're recovering. They range from tasty grilled chicken breasts marinated in herbs and spices to hearty turkey stews simmered with veggies.

There are professional suggestions for cooking methods, seasonings, and serving sizes to make sure that every food is not only tasty but also good for you.

Feel-Good Fish and Seafood Recipes:

Seafood and fish are very good for you, so they are a great choice for people who are healing from mastectomy surgery.

These seafoods are full of minerals, vitamins, and omega-3 fatty acids, which are good for your heart.

They also help with healing and reduce inflammation. Within this part of the mastectomy recovery cookbook, there are many tasty fish and seafood meals that are made to fit a range of tastes and dietary needs.

Every dish, from delicate baked salmon pieces topped with citrus-infused salsa to hearty seafood paellas full of prawns, mussels, and clams, is carefully made to be both healthy and tasty. There are also expert tips on how to choose fresh fish, cook it correctly, and make sure that meals are varied so that people can make smart decisions about their diet after surgery.

Vegetarian and vegan options that are high in nutrients:

Plant-based meals have gotten a lot of attention because they are good for your health in many ways, like lowering your risk of chronic diseases and making you feel better overall.

When recovering from a mastectomy, eating nutrient-dense veggie and vegan foods can give you a lot of the vitamins, minerals, and antioxidants you need to heal and keep your immune system strong. The recipes in this part of the cookbook are all new and tasty ways to show off the variety and richness of plant-based foods.

Each dish, from hearty lentil and veggie stews flavored with fragrant spices to colorful quinoa salads full of protein and fiber, is made to be as healthy as possible without sacrificing taste.

To make sure that vegetarians and vegans get all the nutrients they need after surgery, experts also give tips on how to add iron, calcium, and vitamin B12 to their diets.

The mastectomy recovery cookbook is a complete guide to the best diet after surgery.

It has healing recipes, meal plans, and expert tips for long-term wellness.

The main courses are all healthy, such as tasty chicken and turkey dishes, filling fish and seafood recipes, and nutrient-dense vegetarian and vegan options.

CHAPTER 5

HEALTHY SALADS AND SIDES

Getting enough nutrients is very important for the healing process after surgery. To repair tissues, boost immunity, and promote general health, the body needs a lot of nutrients. In this area, adding healthy sides like veggies and potatoes is very important.

These things not only give you vitamins and minerals that your body needs, but they also make meals more enjoyable, which is important for keeping a good attitude while you're recovering.

In this part, we'll talk about the ideas behind colourful salads, tasty grain and legume sides, and healthy vegetable sides. We'll also talk about their benefits and how they can be used in a diet for mastectomy recovery.

Many different flavors, tastes, and healthy foods can be used in salads, which is why they are so popular. When it comes to healing from a mastectomy, colorful salads are a great way to get a lot of important nutrients, vitamins, and water.

Including different colored veggies like leafy greens, tomatoes, bell peppers, carrots, and cucumbers in your diet helps your body heal by giving it a wide range of vitamins and minerals. Adding protein sources like beans, grilled chicken, salmon, or tofu also makes you feel fuller and helps your body heal itself.

Nuts, seeds, and avocado all have healthy fats, and fruits like berries and citrus pieces make it taste sweet and refreshing. Dressings made from olive oil, vinegar, and herbs not only taste better but also help reduce inflammation. People who are recovering from a mastectomy can enjoy a pleasant, nutrient-dense meal while also improving their health and healing by adding colorful salads to their diet.

Grains and beans are important parts of a healthy diet because they are full of carbs, fiber, protein, and many micronutrients. As you recover from a mastectomy, tasty sides made of grains and legumes can give you long-lasting energy, help your digestive system stay healthy, and speed up the healing process.

Whole grains like brown rice, quinoa, barley, and farro are high in fiber, which makes you feel full and helps your body digest food. Beans, peas, and lentils are all legumes that are high in protein, which is needed to repair muscles and keep the immune system strong.

These foods also have vitamins and antioxidants that fight inflammation and oxidative stress, which are very important for the healing process after surgery.

Adding healthy fats like olive oil or avocado along with flavorful herbs and spices makes grain and bean sides taste better and be healthier. By adding these healthy foods to a person's post-mastectomy recovery diet, they can take care of their bodies while having tasty, filling meals.

Healthy Sides of Vegetables

Because they are full of vitamins, minerals, fiber, and phytonutrients, vegetables are an important part of a healthy diet. Healthy vegetable sides are good for you in many ways, like boosting your immune system, lowering inflammation, and improving gut health.

Cruciferous veggies like broccoli, cauliflower, and Brussels sprouts have chemicals in them that help the body get rid of toxins and may lower the risk of cancer coming back.

This makes them especially good for people who have recently had a mastectomy. Leafy greens like spinach, kale, and Swiss chard are great sources of iron, folate, and vitamins A, C, and K, all of which are needed to repair tissues and make new blood cells. Some root veggies, like beets, carrots, and sweet potatoes, are naturally sweet and full of healthy things like beta-carotene and vitamin C. People recovering from a mastectomy can get the most nutrients out of their food and help their bodies heal by adding a range of colourful vegetables to their side dishes.

CHAPTER 6

SNACKS AND TREATS TO MAKE YOU FEEL BETTER

As you heal from a mastectomy, comforting snacks and treats are very important.

They not only keep you physically healthy, but they also help you feel better emotionally during a tough time.

As part of a post-surgery diet meant to speed up healing, boost energy, and improve overall health, these snacks and treats are important.

This complete guide to the best post-surgery diet for people who have just been diagnosed goes into detail about how important comforting snacks and treats are.

It includes ideas for energizing snacks, healthy treats for treating yourself, and portable snack choices to help your recovery go more smoothly.

After having a mastectomy, it's important to eat snacks that are high in nutrients that will help the body heal and keep you from getting tired. Energizing snacks give you a quick energy boost without giving up any of the nutrients you need. Fresh fruits like oranges, bananas, and apples are great options because they are full of minerals, vitamins, and natural sugars that give you energy right away. Fruits that are eaten with a protein source, like nut butter or Greek yogurt, can make you feel fuller and give you more energy.

Nuts and seeds are also very healthy snacks because they contain healthy fats, protein, and fiber, all of which help keep blood sugar levels steady and give you long-lasting energy. Some very healthy choices are almonds, walnuts, and pumpkin seeds.

Because they are high in healthy fats and complex carbohydrates, whole grain crackers or rice cakes with hummus or avocado can also be a filling and energizing snack.

Energy balls made from nuts, dried fruits, and oats are a quick and healthy option for people who like to make their snacks. You can make these small treats ahead of time without much trouble, and you can change them up by adding things like chia seeds, coconut bits, or dark chocolate chips.

Smoothies and protein shakes are also great choices for a quick and refreshing snack because they contain carbs, protein, and water, all of which help the body heal and replace nutrients that it has lost.

Indulgent treats that are good for you:

It's important to eat nutrient-dense snacks to help your body heal, but enjoying healthy treats can also improve your overall health and happiness during the recovery time. Treats that are good for you are made with healthy ingredients that add flavour and are good for you. Dark chocolate, for instance, is full of antioxidants that may help lower inflammation and boost mood, so you can enjoy it without feeling bad about it.

Whole grain flours are used to make comfort foods like oatmeal cookies and banana bread that don't have a lot of extra sugars or refined carbs.

Natural sweeteners like honey or maple syrup can be used to make these treats sweeter. Nuts, seeds, or dried fruits can be added for extra flavour and texture. Adding things like oats, flaxseeds, and cinnamon to baked goods can also be good for you in other ways, like helping your stomach and keeping your blood sugar levels steady.

If you're wanting something sweet, you can make your own granola bars or trail mix. They are also a quick and easy way to get energy and nutrients. Mixing things like rolled oats, nuts, seeds, and dried fruits together lets people make their snacks that suit their tastes and dietary needs. Also, frozen treats like fruit sorbet or yogurt popsicles are a healthy and refreshing option to regular ice cream. They contain probiotics, minerals, and vitamins that help the immune system and digestive health.

Maintaining a healthy diet while recovering from a mastectomy may require people to have easy-to-carry snacks that they can eat while they're on the go or when they're busy. Snacks that you can take with you should be easy to pack, not go bad, and give you steady energy to help you heal and recover. People can make sure they have healthy snacks available all day by putting together snack packs or grab-and-go packages with a mix of protein, carbs, and healthy fats.

Trail mix, which is a mix of nuts, seeds, dried fruits, and whole grain cereals, is a great snack that you can take with you. It has a good balance of macronutrients and can be changed to fit your tastes. In the same way, protein bars or energy bars made with natural ingredients like nuts, seeds, and dried vegetables are a quick and easy way to get energy and important nutrients while you're on the go. To improve your health and well-being as a whole, choose bars with few added sugars and artificial chemicals.

You can wash and put fresh fruit like apples, grapes, or berries into containers that you can take with you for easy eating during the day.

Fruits that are paired with single servings of nut butter or cheese sticks can make you feel fuller and give you more nutrients. Also, rice cakes or crackers made from whole grains that come with individual amounts of hummus, guacamole, or cheese spread are quick and easy snacks that can be eaten anywhere.

Finally, comforting foods like snacks and treats are very important for getting better after a mastectomy because they give you energy, nutrients, and mental support during a tough time. By adding healthy treats for treats, snack ideas that will get you going, and snack options that you can take with you after surgery, people can help their bodies heal, get their energy back, and stay healthy in the long run. People can make their recovery process more resilient and positive by making conscious choices and putting nourishing ingredients first.

CHAPTER 7

IS ABOUT WATER AND DRINKS.

Making sure you stay hydrated is an important part of recovering from a mastectomy. Staying hydrated is good for your health in general, helps wounds heal, keeps your body temperature stable, and keeps your body working.

Staying hydrated can also help with common problems that come up after surgery, like feeling tired and having trouble going to the toilet.

It's important to think about both the amount and quality of fluids you drink when you're thinking about staying hydrated. Choose drinks that are good for you and keep you hydrated.

These drinks can also help your body heal and improve your general health.

Herbal teas and water with herbs

Drinking infused water or plant tea is a great way to stay hydrated and get extra health benefits.

Adding fruits, veggies, and herbs to water gives it a natural flavor and important nutrients without the sugars and chemicals that are often found in commercial drinks. Infused water can be a healthy and refreshing option to sugary drinks or plain water for people who have recently had a mastectomy. Herbal teas with soothing ingredients like chamomile, ginger, or peppermint can help ease pain after surgery, lower inflammation, and encourage rest. Adding these drinks to your diet after surgery not only helps you stay hydrated but also improves your health and comfort while you're healing.

Recipes for healing smoothies

Smoothies are flexible, nutrient-dense drinks that can be changed to fit different tastes and nutrition needs. These foods are especially good for people who are healing from mastectomy surgery because they are easy to eat, and digest, and are full of nutrients. Adding leafy veggies, fruits, nuts, seeds, and plant-based proteins to smoothie recipes can help your body get the vitamins, minerals, antioxidants, and protein it needs to heal and recover. Smoothies can also be changed to help with certain post-surgery symptoms or nutritional needs, like helping tissues heal, lowering inflammation, or handling digestive problems. Including healing drinks in your diet after surgery makes sure you get enough nutrients and gives you a tasty, easy way to stay hydrated and fed while you're healing.

Drinks that are full of nutrients

Besides water, herbal teas, and smoothies, many other nutrient-dense drinks can help you heal after a mastectomy. Some of these are protein shakes, bone broth, fresh drinks, and coconut water. Juices that have just been squeezed are full of vitamins, minerals, and antioxidants that can help heal tissues, boost the immune system, and improve health in general. Because it is high in electrolytes, coconut water is a great way to replace the vitamins and fluids you lose during surgery or exercise. Collagen, amino acids, minerals, and other nutrients found in bone soup help wounds heal, joints stay healthy, and the gut stay intact.

Making protein shakes with good protein powders like whey, pea, or collagen protein is an easy way to get more protein, which is important for healing muscles and tissues after surgery. Adding these nutrient-dense drinks to a diet after surgery gives people a range of ways to stay hydrated that meet their own nutritional needs and preferences, which helps them recover as quickly as possible and stay healthy in the long run.

staying hydrated is important for healing after a mastectomy, and choosing the right drinks can speed up the process and improve your health in general. For a relaxing and healthy drink, try infused water or herbal tea. For an easy and nutrient-dense way to stay hydrated and healthy, try healing smoothie recipes. Drinks that are high in nutrients, like fresh juices, coconut water, bone broth, and protein shakes, can help your body heal even more by giving you vitamins, minerals, antioxidants, and protein. By including these ways to stay hydrated and drink in a post-surgery diet, people can speed up their healing and set themselves up for long-term health and vitality.

CHAPTER 8
TIPS FOR PLANNING AND MAKING MEALS

Planning and making meals ahead of time are important parts of recovering from a mastectomy because they make sure that people who have had this major surgery get the best diet to help them heal and stay healthy overall. This part will talk about effective ways to plan meals, how to cook and freeze large amounts of food at once, and time-saving meal-making tricks made just for mastectomy healing.

Strategies for Planning Meals That Work

People who are healing from mastectomy surgery need to plan their meals well so that they always have healthy meals without having to stress about making them every day. To begin, it's important to make a flexible meal plan that takes into account personal tastes, dietary needs, and the need to heal. To help your body heal and your immune system, start by eating a wide range of nutrient-dense foods, like lean proteins, whole grains, fruits, and veggies.

When you are first getting better, when digestion may not be working as well, you might want to plan meals that are easy to eat and gentle on the stomach. Focus on eating foods that are high in antioxidants, vitamins, and minerals.

These nutrients are very important for helping tissues heal and lowering inflammation. Aim for a mix of macronutrients as well. Carbohydrates give you energy, protein helps repair tissues, and healthy fats make you feel full and help your body absorb nutrients.

Another good way to plan meals is to cook large amounts of basic foods and meals ahead of time. This saves time and makes sure that healthy meals are always available while the person is recovering. You should pick recipes that are easy to make in big quantities, like soups, stews, casseroles, and grain-based salads.

You can freeze cooked food in portion-sized containers for later use. This makes reheating easy and requires little work on busy days.

You might also want to use online recipe databases, meal-planning apps, and cookbooks that are specifically made for recovering from a mastectomy as tools and resources for food planning. People can get ideas, advice, and help from these sources to make tasty, healthy meals that fit their specific dietary needs and tastes.

people who are recovering from a mastectomy need to plan their meals in a way that makes sure they get the right nutrients to help their healing and general health. People can speed up the meal preparation process and focus on their recovery by eating a variety of nutrient-dense foods, cooking large amounts of basic ingredients at once, and using tools for meal planning.

For people recovering from a mastectomy, batch cooking, and freezing meals are very helpful methods that let them have a steady supply of healthy meals with little work. To get the most out of cooking and saving in bulk, it's important to follow some important rules and tips.

First, pick recipes like soups, stews, casseroles, and pasta meals that can be made in large quantities and frozen. The ingredients in these recipes usually freeze well and don't change the taste or texture when reheated. Also, choose meals that are well-balanced and full of nutrients, like those that have a range of proteins, carbs, and healthy fats to help your body recover and stay healthy.

For freezer burn prevention and food preservation, it's important to buy high-quality storage cases that can go in the freezer and keep food fresh. Before freezing, put cooked meals into containers that are the right size for each person.

This makes it easy to warm and serve as needed.

To keep track of how fresh food is and to avoid throwing it away, write the name of the dish and the date it was made on the containers.

Also, think about using items that can be frozen, like cooked grains, beans, and vegetables, which are easy to add to different recipes and meal combinations. Getting these items ready ahead of time saves time and effort when making meals and makes sure that you always have what you need for healthy, satisfying meals.

Also, make sure you follow food safety rules when you cook and freeze a lot of meals at once. For example, let cooked food cool to room temperature before freezing it, and don't refreeze thawed meals to stop bacteria from growing and spreading sickness. To keep the quality and flavor, thaw frozen meals overnight in the fridge or the warming setting of your microwave.

batch cooking and freezing are helpful skills for people who are healing from mastectomy surgery because they let them have a steady supply of healthy meals without having to cook every day. Individuals can speed up the meal preparation process and focus on their healing by selecting appropriate recipes, purchasing good storage containers, and following food safety rules.

How to Save Time When Making Meals

Meal preparation hacks that save time are important for people recovering from a mastectomy so they can focus on rest and healing while still enjoying tasty and healthy meals. Focusing on making food preparation as quick and easy as possible, these hacks make it easier to stick to a healthy diet while you're recovering.

To save time when making meals, use kitchen gadgets and machines like slow cookers, pressure cookers, and rice cookers.

These can cut down on the time you spend cooking by hand by a large amount.

These gadgets let you cook without having to use your hands. They only need a little direction and work to make tasty, satisfying meals.

Think about buying tools that can do more than one thing when it comes to cooking. This will make the process of making meals even easier.

Using pre-cut and pre-packaged foods, like salad veggies that have already been washed and chopped, and grains and proteins that have already been cooked is another way to save time.

These handy items can cut down on prep time by a lot and make it easier to put together quick, healthy meals with little work. Also, think about buying a lot of frozen fruits and veggies. They are just as healthy as fresh ones, and they last longer, making it easier to add them to meals and recipes.

Also, get into the habit of "planned leftovers" by making bigger amounts of meals on purpose and using the extras to make new dishes throughout the week. For instance, roasted veggies can be added to soups, salads, or grain bowls.

Grains and proteins that are left over can be used to make stir-fries, casseroles, or wraps. This method not only saves time and effort but also cuts down on food waste and makes cooking more fun.

Additionally, you might want to ask family, friends, or carers to help you prepare meals. This way, you can share the work and get support while you're recovering. Giving simple jobs like chopping vegetables, putting together salads, or setting the table for other people will give you more time and energy to rest and recover.

people who are healing from mastectomy surgery need to find ways to make meals faster and easier so they can eat a healthy diet with little effort.

Using cooking tools and appliances, adding convenience foods, looking forward to planned leftovers, and asking for help from others can make preparing meals easier so that people can focus on their healing.

CHAPTER 9

MINDFUL EATING AND HEALTH HABITS

Mindful eating and other wellness practices are very important for getting better after a mastectomy. This detailed guide stresses how important it is to change the way you eat and include healthy activities in your daily life to speed up the healing process. Focusing on nourishing the body with healthy foods and practicing relaxation techniques can help people improve their physical and mental health, creating an environment that is good for recovery.

Why mindful eating is important:

When you eat mindfully, you pay full attention to all of your senses while noticing your thoughts, feelings, and physical cues. This exercise helps people develop a stronger connection with food, which makes them more aware of when they are hungry or full.

Mindful eating is an important way for people who have had a mastectomy to get the best diet and help their bodies heal. People can make smart food choices that include nutrient-dense foods that are important for healing by being aware of what they eat. Mindful eating can also help reduce the stress and anxiety that come with surgery, giving people a sense of control and empowerment over their health path.

Using techniques for relaxation:

It is very important to use relaxation methods to help with healing and overall health after a mastectomy. Mind and body can both relax and feel less stressed with techniques like progressive muscle relaxing, deep breathing exercises, and regular meditation. These activities help ease muscle tension, improve the quality of sleep, and boost happiness, all of which are important for the healing process.

People can lessen the physical and mental effects of surgery by setting aside time every day to relax.

This will make the transition to life after surgery easier. Relaxation techniques also help people deal with the problems and unknowns that may come up during the recovery time, which builds inner strength and resilience.

Self-Care Tips for Health and Happiness:

Self-care includes many different activities that are meant to take care of your mind, body, and spirit. When recovering from a mastectomy, it's important to put yourself first to improve your general health and feel more in control.

This means taking care of your physical, mental, and spiritual needs as a whole when you care for yourself. Some ways to take care of yourself are to do gentle exercises like yoga or tai chi to get stronger and more flexible, to write in a book or be creative as a way to deal with your feelings, and to get help from friends, family, or support groups. Self-care also includes taking care of yourself by eating well and getting enough rest, which helps the body heal and recover.

People can improve their resilience and keep a good attitude on their recovery journey by making self-care regular parts of their lives.

mindful eating and other wellness practices are important parts of recovering from a mastectomy because they help with healing and overall health in the long term.

By adopting mindful eating habits, learning how to relax, and putting self-care first, people can handle the challenges of life after surgery with more ease and strength. This complete guide gives helpful information and useful tips on how to apply these practices in everyday life, giving people who have had mastectomy surgery the power to regain their health and vitality.

CHAPTER 10

IS ABOUT SUPPORT RESOURCES AND EXTRA INFORMATION

Having access to support groups and extra information can make the process of recovering from a mastectomy a lot easier, both physically and emotionally. This part is a complete list of all the resources that are out there. It has contact information for support groups, suggested reading and resources, and answers to frequently asked questions (FAQs). The goal of these resources is to give patients the support, information, and direction they need to make it through their recovery journey successfully.

How to Get in Touch with Support Groups:

Support groups are very important for people recovering from a mastectomy because they give them emotional support, encouragement, and a sense of community.

These groups usually have other patients, survivors, carers, and healthcare workers who understand the problems and worries that come with getting better. You can get the contact information for local and online support groups at hospitals, cancer centers, community groups, or websites that are just for breast cancer support. People who have had a mastectomy can feel safe in these groups where they can talk about their experiences, get advice, and learn useful ways to deal with the physical and emotional parts of recovery.

Reading suggestions and links:

To speed up the healing process, it's important to learn about mastectomy recovery, nutrition, and general health. Many books, articles, websites, and other educational materials can help patients and their caretakers learn useful things and get useful tips. Some books that may be suggested for reading are those written by nutritionists, doctors who specialize in breast cancer care, and people who have had a mastectomy. Also, trustworthy online sources like medical websites, forums, and support platforms have a lot of information on a wide range of topics, from getting ready for surgery to getting care afterward and planning for long-term wellness. These resources give patients the information they need to make smart choices about their recovery and start living in a way that helps them heal and be healthy.

FAQs, or Frequently Asked Questions, are:

People who have had a mastectomy often have questions and concerns about different parts of their treatment, recovery, and daily life. Answering these frequently asked questions (FAQs) can help reduce stress, make things clearer, and make the recovery process go more smoothly.

Some of the most common questions are about how to deal with pain after surgery, how to care for wounds, how much exercise is okay, what foods to eat, how to get emotional support, and what complications might happen. Healthcare professionals, support groups, and online resources often put together lists of frequently asked questions (FAQs) and answer them in detail based on patient experiences and practices that have been shown to work.

Taking care of these common worries can help patients feel more confident and in control as they go through each stage of their recovery.

having access to support groups and extra information is very helpful for people recovering from a mastectomy. These resources help patients feel more in control of their recovery, learn more about it, and improve their overall health.

They can do this by connecting with support groups, reading suggested books, or looking for answers to frequently asked questions.

Patients can get through their recovery with confidence, strength, and hope if they know how to use these resources well.

CONCLUSION

Focusing on good nutrition during the time after surgery is very important for speeding up recovery and promoting long-term health.

This complete guide has talked about many different aspects of making a healing diet, from understanding what nutrients you need while you're recovering to making sure you have all the ingredients and tools you need in your kitchen.

We looked at a lot of healing recipes that are good for different meal times, so you can have a healthy journey from breakfast to snacks and drinks.

The focus on healthy ingredients, mindful eating, and efficient meal planning shows how important it is to take care of your whole health while you're recovering.

Each recipe, from energizing smoothies to hearty soups, tasty main courses, and colourful salads, is made to provide essential nutrients and accommodate a range of dietary needs, including vegetarian and vegan options. We've also talked about how important it is to stay hydrated and given you some refreshing drink options to keep you hydrated and energized all day.

In addition to talking about diet, this guide has also talked about how important it is to eat mindfully, use relaxation techniques, and take care of yourself for your overall health.

We've also given you access to helpful resources and information about support groups to help you on your way to recovery.

If you follow the ideas in this guide and add healing recipes, meal plans, and professional advice to your routine after surgery, you can speed up your recovery and start a path to long-term health. Remember that feeding your body is not only an important part of healing but also a key part of keeping your health and vitality in general.

You can confidently get through the time after surgery with hard work, mindfulness, and the help of this complete guide. This will make the transition to a healthier, happier future go more smoothly.

www.ingramcontent.com/pod-product-compliance
Lightning Source LLC
Chambersburg PA
CBHW070316290526
45791CB00003B/1134